Counseling Interac Traumatically Brain Injured Clients

Keith D. Cicerone, Ph.D.

Clinical Director, Center for Head Injuries
JFK-Johnson Rehabilitation Institute
Edison, New Jersey 08820

Consulting Neuropsychologist
Trauma Section, Department of Surgery
Robert Wood Johnson University Hospital
New Brunswick, New Jersey

Associate Professor of
Physical Medicine and Rehabilitation
University of Medicine and Dentistry of New Jersey-
Robert Wood Johnson Medical School
Piscataway, New Jersey

**Robert T. Fraser, Ph.D. and
David C. Clemmons, Ph.D.**
EDITORS

**Supported by the office of Special Education and
Rehabilitative Services
Grant#HI129T80031-89**

S_L^t

St. Lucie Press
Boca Raton   Boston   London   New York   Washington, D.C.

TABLE OF CONTENTS

Introduction

Traumatic brain injury represents a tremendous obstacle to effective functioning for clients, and this is very often expressed through their difficulty and frustration around the issue of return to work. This is not surprising in our culture and society, since the inability to return to work carries both social and economic costs, and notions of *recovery of function* and *being normal* are associated (rightly or wrongly) with return to work. Not only clients and family members, but also rehabilitation therapists, counselors, and funding agencies often see return to work as the sign-post of successful rehabilitation and recovery after traumatic brain injury.

Price and Baumann (1990) point out that working is often considered the key to normalization after a traumatic brain injury, since many of these clients have already established normal developmental milestones including personal and career decisions.

Thus, the traumatic injury interferes with a lifelong process through which the individual was establishing a personal identity and social role. The injury, and particularly the inability to work, thereby disrupts the individual's sense of purpose, productivity and self-worth. The inability to work may have far-reaching consequences for a person's capacity for autonomous functioning. For this reason, the central concern of the counseling process can be seen as one of assisting a person to re-establish a satisfactory level of *personal and functional sufficiency*. We use the concept of personal sufficiency to refer to a person's ability to function and achieve goals with various levels of assistance or reliance on others, and with the aim of acknowledging a need for interdependence.

With respect to vocational counseling, an emphasis may be placed on fostering the client's ability to make choices, facilitating a sense of self-determination, and providing him* with the appropriate resources. This can often involve allowing the client to make decisions with which the therapist or counselor does not agree, or which in fact appear to be unrealistic. Unlike the client with a history of developmental disability, the traumatically injured client is forced to re-align expectancies for future functioning despite having a personal history of career decisions

---

* Where necessary, we have replaced the plural pronoun "their" with the singular, masculine pronoun "him" and its derivative "his" in order to facilitate grammatically correct sentences, allowing the pronoun to agree in number with the noun it replaces. The words "him" and "his" are therefore not used here to denote gender.

and achievement. Clients will often respond negatively to the suggestion that they will be unable to attain 100% of their pre-injury status, and cling stubbornly to their aspirations even when faced with repeated, objective evidence to the contrary. The emotional responses to this confrontation can include depression, catastrophic anxiety, minimization of deficits, devaluation of the therapist and therapy, and seemingly contradictory risk-taking behaviors which jeopardize their stated goals.

In addition, consequences of the brain injury often include an altered capacity for "insight", a reduced ability to identify the sources of one's own distress, or difficulty in recognizing, understanding or anticipating the consequences of one's own behavior. Thus, in order to be effective, counseling must not only facilitate the person's capacity for self-determination in the face of external barriers, but also help the client gain access to and awareness of the inner psychological processes which influence their decisions. In this regard, counseling and psychotherapy with a client having a traumatic brain injury is no different from any other. It does require, however, that the counselor understand the various ways in which the traumatic brain injury may be manifested and the common cognitive, emotional and personality disturbances which can occur.

Psychological Disturbances after Traumatic Brain Injury

The discussion of psychological disturbances after traumatic brain injury will include changes in thinking, feeling or behaving that influence the person's ability to function as well as his self-image and self-esteem. Prigatano (1986) and others have suggested that psychological disturbances after brain injury can be classified according to three categories. The first consists of neuropsychologically mediated problems which arise as a direct consequence of organic damage. The second category consists of emotionally based problems that are related to a reaction to the injury or attempts to cope with the effects of the injury. The third category consists of pre-injury personality characteristics which may persist after injury, and influence both the expression of neurologic damage and the person's reactions to injury.

Neuropsychologically Mediated and Organic Problems

In general, there appears to be a fairly consistent association between neurologically-based personality and behavioral symptoms and the severity of injury. These symptoms may be especially prominent during the early stage of recovery and coincide with the period of cognitive disorganization. For example, it is not uncommon for hospitalized clients to become extremely agitated and even combative once they have begun emerging from coma. This probably represents a period in which a person is more responsive to various sources of stimulation in his or her environment, yet still lacks the cognitive ability to either filter out irrelevant stimulation or make complete sense of their surroundings. The agitation may be accompanied by gross misunderstandings or distortions of what is going on around them, as well as apparently bizarre interpretations in an attempt to make sense of their environment. At this stage, it is not unusual for the person to misidentify the hospital as a hotel, or to believe that they are at work. This may coincide with a period of post-traumatic amnesia, in which the person's ability to recall information from moment to moment is dramatically reduced, so that older and more familiar memories are more easily recalled and will "intrude" on current events. Thus, it is the combination of direct changes in the functioning of nervous tissue and the accompanying cognitive limitations that underlie this type of psychological disturbance, and it can be important to recognize these behaviors as neuropsychologically based confabulations or misperceptions rather than as any form of psychiatric disturbance.

This same combination of neurologic and cognitive components can be seen with more persisting behavioral abnormalities. For example, clients may have difficulty controlling their temper or experience periodic anger outbursts. Frequently, there will appear to be minimal or no provocation for these episodes. Yet they probably represent, once again, a *reduced tolerance* for levels of stimulation which had previously been tolerated, along with the *disinhibition* and the full release of an accompanying emotional response. Even in cases of relatively mild traumatic brain injury, an increase in irritability and loss of patience are among the personality changes most commonly reported by clients and (especially) by family members.

In many cases, the degree of psychological and behavioral disturbance appears to be related to the overall degree of injury and the extent of neurologic damage. This may be particularly true with head trauma, in which the diffuse disruption of nerve fibers extending throughout the brain is one of the primary mechanisms of injury. There are also behavioral abnormalities, however, which may be related to particularly focal areas of injury. In traumatic brain injury, both the frontal and the anterior temporal lobes are particularly susceptible to contusion due to the bony structure of the skull in these areas. Both the frontal and temporal lobes are known to regulate various types of socially-appropriate behaviors and emotional reactions, so that damage to one or both of these areas may again increase the potential for neurologically mediated behavior problems or personality changes.

Pepping and Roueche (1990) have summarized many of the personality and cognitive changes which may result from neurologic damage. Among the personality changes considered to be organically based are the following:

1. Egocentricity and loss of ability to show empathy (frontal)
2. Poor social judgement, impulsive or inappropriate social behavior (frontal)
3. Disinhibition of emotional reactions, thoughts, or actions (frontal)
4. Loss of the self-critical attitude (frontal)
5. Childish or silly behaviors, euphoria (frontal)
6. Apathy, lack of concern, and lack of motivation
7. Emotional lability, mood swings, inappropriate laughing or crying (frontal, temporal, frontotemporal)
8. Increased irritability and aggression (temporal)
9. Suspiciousness, paranoia, misperception of the intentions of others (temporal, parietal)
10. Catastrophic reactions (frontal, temporal, diffuse)

When considering possible neuropsychologically mediated behavior problems, it is also important to recognize the contribution of cognitive deficits. Among the most common deficits after traumatic brain injury are reduced attention and concentration and heightened distractibility. This may result in difficulty in following instructions or learning new information; probably more importantly, the client may look as if he or she is "not paying attention" despite repeated requests to do so. Attentional deficits are likely to be most prominent when the client is required to pay attention to more than one thing at a time. This may prove impossible to do, although the client is capable of performing each activity one at a time.

Memory problems are also particularly prominent, and are among the symptoms most likely to be identified by clients and their families as presenting problems. Reduced learning ability and poor memory are among the principal problems associated with poor work performance, as will be discussed more fully below. Not only may they interfere with the acquisition of job skills, but they can also result in "poor" work behaviors. We have been notified of clients who failed to return from a lunch break because they forgot that they were at work!

Difficulty with "executive" functioning such as reduced initiation and persistence on a task, poor planning ability, reduced organization and difficulty correcting errors are frequently a consequence of traumatic brain injury. These deficits will obviously interfere with a person's ability to function without supervision. It is not uncommon to see a dissociation between a client's intact ability to *verbally describe* a procedure or appropriate social response and their impaired ability to *actually perform* the required response. Not surprisingly, this can create the impression that the client is simply unwilling to respond appropriately or that they are noncompliant.

Emotional Reactions to Injury

Emotional reactions after injury appear to be particularly related to the recognition of reduced competencies, and more generally, a sense of loss of self. Unlike the neurologically mediated problems, emotional reactions appear to bear no consistent relation to the neurologic severity of injury. In addition, the degree of emotional distress and difficulty adjusting to the effects of the injury frequently increase over time. During the acute period, there may be little evidence that clients are experiencing any emotional distress although their behavior is inappropriate and disorganized; in fact, there may be little awareness of difficulty. As the client experiences repeated or prolonged difficulty, or as it becomes apparent that the extent of recovery of work or social functioning is not going to be as great as expected or hoped for, emotional reactions may worsen.

Depression is a common reaction to the losses sustained by the person with a traumatic brain injury. Increases in cognitive ability and self-awareness over time may be accompanied by increased recognition of deficits, and increasing depression. The attempt to return to work may be the first time that the client really confronts the discrepancies between his or her current level of functioning and pre-injury abilities. It is not uncommon to see a period of elation on returning to work, followed by increasing sadness and disappointment. The most significant symptoms of a clinical depression are subjective feelings of sadness and depressed mood, and the loss of interest or pleasure in usual activities. Additional symptoms include poor appetite or overeating, sleep disturbance, fatigue or lack of energy, low self esteem, feelings of worthlessness, excessive guilt, and difficulty concentrating or making decisions. Anxiety, while probably less prominent than depression, may be particularly evident in clients attempting to avoid "detection" of their deficits or embarrassment. There may be an avoidance of the work setting, or other people in the work setting. Feelings of mistrust, isolation, and social withdrawal may become prominent if the anxiety persists.

In general, fluctuations in a client's emotional reactions to injury are not uncommon as they experience varying degrees of adjustment and awareness. These changes are also accompanied by, and influenced by changes in the level of acceptance, understanding and tolerance exhibited by family, friends, employers and others.

Pre-injury Personality Characteristics

Pre-injury personality characteristics may be exaggerated after injury; other clients may show drastic alterations or reversals of their personality traits. It is important to obtain information and an adequate understanding of a person's premorbid functioning before attributing changes in behavior to the effects of the injury. We have frequently started to treat patients for varying behavioral "abnormalities" only to discover with further exploration that this was probably not very different from their pre-injury functioning. The client's coping style and responses to stressful situations before the injury needs to be explored. Tendencies toward minimization or amplification of emotional situations, adaptability to change, willingness to consider psychological explanations for one's behavior, and tolerance for interpersonal disclosure are all likely to be carried over and influence the person's response to injury and to treatment.

Similarly, family relationships, including the need for affiliation and level of dependency within the family system will influence treatment. We have found it helpful to examine at least two dimensions of family functioning. First, the degree to which the family system considers itself responsible (or at fault) for the client's disability. Second, the degree to which the family system holds itself accountable for the client's future.

Social functioning and status need to be considered. Various forms of risk-taking and sensation-seeking, as well as substance use or abuse, may be common among the persons at greatest risk to sustain a traumatic brain injury.

In general, pre-existing personality, coping, family, and socialization factors probably represent respective limitations, although not necessarily contra-indications, to therapy.

Psychological Assessment

An important responsibility of the counselor working with clients who have traumatic brain injury, is the recognition and differentiation among these various psychological disturbances. Obviously, differing combinations of organic, emotional and characterological disorders may exist, and at times it may not be possible to isolate any single component. However, familiarity with the various possible presentations will increase the likelihood of an appropriate therapeutic intervention. For example, a 35-year-old man was referred for a psychological evaluation by his rehabilitation counselor for evaluation of depression and possible malingering. The client had sustained a closed head injury two and one-half years earlier, and although he had been severely injured, he had made good neurologic recovery and had been discharged from the hospital after two months with "no apparent deficits." He then returned to his job as a loan officer, but was unable to follow through with any previous accounts and was temporarily assigned to assist another bank officer. However, he continued to repeatedly enter his old office, manipulate his old accounts, and generally behave as if he had never been absent from his job, despite being told several times not to do so. Shortly after, he was given a medical leave of absence and recommended for a psychiatric evaluation. He did see a psychiatrist (although he did not understand the reason for the referral, he complied in order to not lose his job) who diagnosed a "depression with psychomotor retardation" and placed him on anti-depressant medication. He had been unable to return to work since that time. Although he attempted to do so on several occasions, he would become disruptive and verbally insulting to his supervisors, and he was then eventually released.

On the psychological evaluation, he stated that he would still like to return to his former job, and still thought he would be able to do so with no difficulty. With direct questioning he admitted to having some memory problems which might limit his ability to former work, but when asked to name three other jobs he would like to do he could only suggest becoming a supervisor at his former bank. When questioned about the impact of his injury on his daily functioning, he again acknowledged some forgetfulness, with an apparent lack of concern. He spent his time watching television and did little else around the house, neglecting home maintenance activities and his former hobby as a locksmith. When questioned about this, he stated that he still enjoyed his hobby, but all his equipment was downstairs in the basement and although he was physically able to walk downstairs he "preferred not to." His wife reported that he used to be very outgoing, but now rarely interacted with family or friends. He had become much more compliant in acquiescing to her suggestions or preferences, and he was less motivated and rarely initiated or followed through on any action on his own. Although usually withdrawn since the injury, he had had several verbal outbursts lasting several minutes, after which he was either very remorseful or denied that the incident had even occurred. He had little understanding of why he had been let go from his work, did not recall any inappropriate behaviors or conflicts with his supervisors, and in general saw no reason why he could not return to work at any time.

While this man exhibited no depressed mood or loss of interests, he certainly had a reduced awareness of his deficits and an inability to recognize the impact of his social behaviors, as well as a general reduction in activity level and initiation. He had never appreciated that he was unable to perform his prior job, and in his mind had been subjected to repeated, senseless changes and frustrations. With a program of education regarding his neurologic injury and neuropsychological deficits, counseling to assist him identify aspects of his behavior which were different from his prior self (including the effect of his memory deficits on work and daily functioning), and perhaps most importantly a structured, consistent system of behavioral supervision (both at home and at the bank) he was able to return to employment. It still remained necessary for him to work at a much reduced capacity. While intervention did not, certainly, alleviate this man's neurologic and cognitive disability, he was able to improve his daily functioning, once his behaviors were understood in terms of a neurologically mediated disturbance, rather than either an emotional or volitional disorder.

Counseling Interactions and the Therapeutic Relationship

Basic Interaction Considerations

While neuropsychologically mediated deficits exhibit a fairly consistent though modest relationship to clients' everyday functioning and employment capabilities, personality and emotional factors exert a significant influence, at least on clients' subjective disability. Chelune, Heaton, and Lehman (1986) found that clients' complaints of cognitive, memory, communication and sensorimotor impairments were more strongly related to the results from the Minnesota Multiphasic Personality Inventory than to their neuropsychological test performance. In particular, the clients' levels of emotional distress discriminated between those who "exaggerated" and those who "minimized" their disability, irrespective of actual neuropsychological impairment based on test results. Changes in levels of emotional distress over the course of brain injury rehabilitation appear to vary according to clients' subjective reports of disability and can be related to rehabilitation outcomes (employment status), independent of changes in neuropsychological impairment (Fordyce & Roueche, 1986). On the basis of these studies, it is likely that clients' emotional and personality status will influence their ability to function in everyday life and their ability to return to successful employment, whatever the clients' work skills and level of ability may be. These factors therefore need to be considered within the context of any counseling or therapeutic approach.

In addition to the potential impact of cognitive deficits on daily living and vocational functioning, these impairments will influence the nature and success of therapeutic interactions. Given the emphasis on verbal interaction and self-observation characteristic of many counseling therapies, deficits in language and self-awareness require specific consideration. Clients frequently will have difficulty with complex language, with abstract language, and with the use of metaphor. This is not limited to clients who are frankly (or even subtly) aphasic, but may be secondary to problems with attending to lengthy or complex conversation; remembering difficult or abstract prose material; or with higher-level reasoning. Basic considerations for the counselor include the reliance on simple sentence structure; the avoidance of overly long statements; the use of specific examples; and remaining sensitive to the client's level of understanding. It is not effective to rely on a client's facial expression or body language to gauge his understanding, since this may not be accurate. Confused by unnecessarily complex, abstract or metaphorical language, the client may add to the confusion by giving nonverbal or verbal indicators that he understands the content of the language when in fact he is totally "missing the boat." All too frequently, clients exhibit an altogether concrete interpretation of metaphorical language ("well, if you miss the boat, you might not get out of here, or you could be late coming home") or an inability to extract meaning from complex language (e.g., compound sentences, sentences which convey more than one meaning or sentences which carry many pieces of information). It is useful to have the client paraphrase the therapist's statements at different points in the interaction to insure that he understands the meaning and the intent of the communication.

Clients with reduced self-awareness may not understand the nature or the counseling relationship, and may be likely to misinterpret the therapist's intentions. Clients may be unable to understand the meaning of the therapist's interventions or to relate these interventions to their own situation. There may be little appreciation for the way in which their deficits affect their functioning, and so they may not see the reason for being in treatment. This may be mistaken for lack of concern or motivation, when in fact it would be more accurately considered a lack of awareness. Development of the capacity for self-observation may itself be a primary goal of psychotherapy after traumatic brain injury (Cicerone, 1989).

In general, therapeutic interactions should not rely solely on verbal interventions. For example, modeling of behaviors by the therapist and rehearsal of behaviors by the client can usually be incorporated into the therapy interaction without difficulty. These behavioral interventions help to monitor clients' comprehension and ability to take the message outside of the therapy room.

The role of the "therapeutic alliance" has been recognized as a crucial key to change in diverse forms of therapy, but has been given remarkably little attention in the rehabilitation of clients with traumatic brain injury. The therapeutic alliance has three basic characteristics: *client-therapist expectancies* and belief in the helping relationship, *client-therapist collaboration* on the goals and tasks of therapy, and *client commitment* especially as expressed through defensiveness and resistance to treatment.

Client - Therapist Expectancies

The establishment of a common expectation and the initial conceptualization of treatment is an essential aspect of the counselling process. One of the most important aspects of the counseling relationship is to provide clients with a framework to explore the notions of illness and health, normality and disability. The treatment should provide clients with a rationale for their "illness behavior" and enable them to make sense of their symptoms. The initial phases of counseling may be largely didactic, dealing with issues of structural damage to the brain and permanent loss of function, and providing realistic estimates of the clients' future, without precluding the possibility of change and taking away the clients' hope and motivation. The therapist may need to address issues of not only "what has happened to me?' but also "why has this happened to me?" (Prigatano, 1986).

Clients and therapists alike bring with them into the relationship various attributions regarding past performance and treatment possibilities. Clients may tend to underestimate their deficits (Fordyce & Roueche, 1986) while clinicians may tend to overdiagnose pathology (Faust, Guilmette, Hart, Aikes, Fishburne, & Davey, 1988).

The rehabilitation process may generate additional attributions regarding patient change. We have periodically surveyed clients and therapists involved in a brain injury rehabilitation program regarding their beliefs about the reasons for patient improvement, or lack of improvement, in therapy (Cicerone, 1987). Both rehabilitation clients and therapist appear to identify client variables, - that is, the clients' cognitive, emotional and physical deficits - as the primary obstacle to clients' resuming their pre-injury level of functioning. However, among these types of deficits, differences emerge between clients' and therapists' views. Clients are much more likely to attribute their problems to residual physical deficits, and generally minimize the impact of their cognitive deficits. This appears to be a rather robust belief. Clients expressed this opinion whether they were rating themselves, other clients with whom they were familiar, or a prototypical client with a head injury. In addition, there was no relationship between clients' own level of neuropsychological impairment and their tendency to attribute importance to physical rather than cognitive factors. (Emotional factors were considered slightly more important than cognitive factors; this appeared to be particularly true for clients who were further post-injury.) Therapists, on the other hand, gave much greater emphasis to the clients' residual cognitive deficits as reasons for their disability, while generally minimizing their physical deficits. This was true for all disciplines. (Interestingly, emotional factors were this time considered

15

slightly more important than physical factors, and less important than the clients themselves rated them.)

Among therapy variables, the differences in attributions of success and failure are perhaps more striking. Therapists appear to attribute clients' improvement to the therapy, while they attribute lack of progress to the clients' lack of motivation or maintaining unrealistic expectations. Clients are more likely to attribute gains to their own motivation, as well as to the support of family members. They cite the lack of appropriate therapy, not receiving enough therapy, and inadequacy of social support systems as reasons for their lack of improvement. In general, it appears that both clients and therapists attribute success to things over which they have control, and they attribute failure to factors beyond their control.

It is likely that these client-therapist expectancies exert significant influence over the therapeutic process, and may in themselves be important determinants of success and failure. It therefore appears to be important to align client-therapist expectancies throughout treatment. This process should begin during the initial interview with the client, in order to determine what the client expects from treatment and to clarify what the therapist believes himself or herself to be able to provide. The client should also be encouraged to be open about any preconceptions of the process of therapy, and these issues can be acknowledged and addressed directly. At the same time, possible resistances to the treatment can begin to be anticipated.

Various procedures can be utilized to better engage and prepare the client for therapy. Those procedures that attempt to alter the client's expectations to match the therapy are referred to as *role induction* procedures (Beutler & Clarkin, 1990). In general, role induction procedures include efforts to prepare the client for therapy and include three types of interventions: instructional methods, observational and participatory learning, and treatment contracting.

Instructional methods of role induction include written and verbal information about the nature of therapy or the counseling interaction and descriptions of various behaviors which might be expected from the client. These might include the number and frequency of sessions; the length and type of service; the conditions leading to discharge; the nature and frequency of homework assignments; the types of behaviors which the therapist may address (e.g., emotional symptoms, social skills, "unrealistic" expectations) and the types of behaviors expected from the client (e.g., self-disclosure, consideration of alternative career choices, unpaid volunteer work). This type of intervention appears to be especially suited for clients for whom an initial resistance to treatment might be expected to compromise their full understanding of and participation in the counseling process.

Observational and participatory learning procedures allow the client to "practice" the role in therapy outside of the actual treatment. One form of this might be to have clients observe a group session without being required to participate, or to provide the client the opportunity to talk to another client about their experience in therapy. This is not that different from the use of group therapy to allow clients the chance to share their experiences and overcome their sense of isolation through the group involvement, except that it is used as a means of preparing the client for treatment. Another participatory learning procedure is to provide the client with the opportunity to meet with someone other than the counselor every three or four sessions, in order to discuss relationship problems that may arise during therapy. The goal of this intervention is to provide clients with information, suggestions and reinforcement which can enable them to address the problems within their therapy session. This procedure can assist in maintaining their engagement in counseling. The use of observational and participatory learning procedures may be of particular value for clients with significant cognitive impairments. In some cases, this will allow the counselor to provide services to clients who would otherwise be unable to participate in counseling. Since therapy engagement would be generally unlikely for many individuals with pre-existing personality disorders, approaches such as these may also help to attract or retain these types of clients into therapy.

Therapeutic contracting has been widely used in counseling and psychotherapy and is typically successful in attempting to maintain compliance and reduce client drop-out. When used in this manner, the goal is to provide the client with a framework that enables him to make explicit the expectations for treatment and prepare him for treatment, rather than prescribing specific forms of behavior change. Most often, this will involve the establishment of a specific treatment goal or a time-limited course of therapy. The use of time-limited therapy contracting often increases the probability that clients will complete their course of treatment. A serendipitous finding from time-limited therapy is that on average these clients remain in treatment for longer periods of time than do clients in open-ended therapy (Beutler & Clarkin, 1990). Therapeutic contracting should typically include the following components:

1. The time-limits of treatment should be specified. This limit may include a provision for extension or renewal based upon the review of the effectiveness of treatment.

2. The goals of treatment to be accomplished during the time period should be specified, even when it is expected that these may change over the course of the treatment.
3. The contract should represent the expected roles and behaviors of the therapist as well as the expected roles of the client.
4. The consequences of failing to comply with the contract should be specified.
5. The treatment contract may be written out and signed by both parties, in order to maintain a focus on the conditions of treatment and refer back to as necessary.

In using therapeutic contracts with clients with brain injuries, we have found it to be particularly useful in those cases where the complexity of the client's situation or the tendency of the client to incorporate multiple foci into treatment threatens to forestall any appreciable progress. For example, one 28-year-old woman had sustained a severe traumatic brain injury 11 years earlier, and continued to have significant physical and behavioral limitations as well as frequent seizures which prevented her from working consistently or living alone. The seizures required continual medical supervision, but they continued and were a source of social embarrassment to her. She had not been allowed to leave home and live on her own as would have been age-appropriate behavior, which increased her sense of dependency and resentment towards her parents. This had led to multiple episodes of "running away", alcohol abuse and sexual promiscuity, and two prior suicide attempts. She had received several courses of cognitive and vocational rehabilitation and had several supported employment placements. She had initially done well on each of these until an episode of seizures or behavioral dyscontrol occurred. As various issues were addressed in treatment, the client appeared to shift the focus of her complaints to another area. This not only prevented therapy from adequately addressing her various problems, but also reinforced the view that her situation was hopeless. Contracting in this case was effective in negotiating priorities with her, establishing a hierarchical treatment plan and timetable, and in getting this client to agree to see each problem through to some form of resolution.

We have also found the therapeutic contract to be useful when working with clients who have relatively mild residual deficits, and who have already been through at least one course of appropriate therapy, yet who seek to make further change. In these cases, the use of a time-limited contract serves several functions: it allows the chance to promote further gains when the chance of doing so is really rather limited; it makes explicit the expectation that substantial change is unlikely; it

18

removes the onus of failure from both client and therapist, if in fact change does not occur; it allows the therapist to reframe the client's expectation, i.e., "Now I can assure myself that I've made every effort to improve to my maximum potential, and I'm ready to move on as I am." A therapeutic contract may also be applied within an individual treatment session, in order to maintain a focus on a specific goal within that session.

While we have referred to these procedures as methods to alter clients' expectancies, in reality they are also methods which require therapists to adjust expectations and adapt the treatment process to meet clients' needs and ability to utilize therapy. The essence of the client-therapist relationship is the client's belief in the therapist's ability and desire to help.

Dunbar (1980) has noted that therapist behaviors such as "hurried-ness, interruptions, lack of time for listening, inattentiveness, and not identifying the patients problems from the patient's own perspective, will interfere with the therapist's approachability" (p. 80) and limit the therapist's effectiveness. In working with a client with a brain injury who may have specific issues related to the injury, disability, and treatment, the therapist needs to demonstrate his or her understanding and acceptance of the client. One should be able to discuss with clients the neurologic, cognitive and social aspects of their condition. The therapist needs to understand the "traumatic" nature of the injury, and the sudden and irreversible disjunction of the present condition from the pre-injury situation.

Clients with brain injury need to be accepted for who they are as well as for who they may become. Because of their cognitive limitations, interventions may need to be repeated regularly and may seem to be delivered without any effect. This can tempt the therapist to underesti-mate or even abandon the relationship; we have been frequently im-pressed, however, by the emotional impact the relationship has carried in the absence of overt acknowledgments by the client. In fact, the establishment and maintenance of an interpersonal relationship despite the client's physical, cognitive and social limitations is of tremendous importance to the client with a brain injury.

Client - Therapist Collaboration

The formation of an effective client - therapist collaboration relies on the therapist's ability to create a shared understanding and conceptual-ization of therapy, and to negotiate common goals and treatment objectives. In a general rehabilitation setting, the practice of patient and therapist sharing decisions about treatment was more important than interpersonal or affective dimensions of the therapy relationship for the achievement of rehabilitation goals (Lobitz & Shephard, 1983). In a large vocational rehabilitation agency which served a wide variety of patients with neuropsychiatric disabilities, Galano (1977) compared clients for whom no explicit treatment goals were developed, clients who had specific treatment goals determined by their therapist, and clients who actively collaborated with their therapists on the development of their treatment goals. Only active collaboration between therapist and clients on treatment goals resulted in an improvement in the number of treatment goals met or surpassed, and this improvement was not due to differences in the quality or difficulty of the goals established.

In working with clients after brain injury, the ability to form an active-collaborative relationship appears to depend on several client characteristics. These include the organic bases of awareness; severity of cognitive impairments and cognitive disorganization; motivation and behavioral capacity to actively participate in therapy; level of psychological distress; and defensiveness and need to exert control. There are various actions that the therapist can take to address these issues and facilitate the collaborative relationship.

Difficulties in awareness which result from neurologic injury may be persisting limitations which limit the client's ability to apply compensations or participate in therapy (Crosson, Barco, Velozo, Bolesta, Cooper, & Werts, 1989). Crosson et al. have described three types and levels of awareness deficits which may result from brain injury. *Intellectual awareness* is the ability to understand at some level that a particular disability exists. At the simplest level, the client may recognize or acknowledge that something is difficult for them. At another level, the client may be able to identify a number of activities which are difficult and recognize the similarities among them. A higher level of intellectual awareness "is required to recognize the implications of one's deficits, for example, that visuospatial deficits might hamper a career in graphic design." (Crosson et al., 1989).

Clients who are able to describe their deficits, yet fail to see the implications of these same impairments for returning to work, may be particularly frustrating. They can appear to be stubborn or uncooperative in therapy. It is therefore important to understand that this may represent different levels of intellectual awareness.

Intellectual awareness serves as the basis for two further types of awareness. *Emergent awareness* is the ability of a client to recognize a problem while it is actually occurring. *Anticipatory awareness* is the ability to foresee that a problem is likely to occur under certain circumstances because of a deficit. Once again, the therapist needs to be able to understand the possible independence between lower and high levels of awareness. For example, the bank loan officer could eventually describe how his memory deficits and calculation difficulties would prevent him from making certain necessary computations (thus showing intellectual awareness), yet he repeatedly attempted to open new files requiring these very computations whenever he returned to his work (an emergent awareness deficit). *Organic awareness* deficits are probably related to various cognitive impairments.

Cognitive impairments may also limit the client's ability to antici-pate treatment goals and directions or to understand the relationship between the treatment content and the client's own desires. Goal setting should therefore be specific, tangible and concrete. **Several guidelines for setting treatment goals** are appropriate for these clients:

1. **Establish a well-defined treatment focus**. Many clients with head injury and certainly those who exhibit any significant degree of cognitive disorganization will have difficulty appreciating vague or abstract treatment objectives. Treatment goals should be clearly speci-fied and tied to specific behaviors expected from the client. Thus, it is almost always preferable to maintain a focus on specific, behavioral target symptoms rather than complex interpersonal or personality dynamics. Clients may also benefit from being given a choice between a limited number of treatment goals, rather than leaving this open ended. This enlists them in the process of making relevant treatment decisions while reducing the level of cognitive complexity.

2. **Set proximal goals**. It is easier to maintain focus on a goal which the client can attain within a reasonable amount of time and receive direct concrete feedback. For example, setting a goal of" completing four out of five math problems correctly this week" may be more effective in maintaining the client's involvement and participation than the goal of balancing the checkbook for the month or completing a math course.

3. **Use mediating goals**. The relationship between the proximal goals and the eventual functional ability should be made explicit. These can be conceptualized as the steps required to move the client from his current status to achievement of a desired outcome.

4. **Use comprehension checks**. The client's understanding of the reason for a given activity or intervention should be monitored by having the client repeat or paraphrase this information. This should be done at least every session or every time a new goal or activity is estab-lished. Written information can be provided, or graphic charts and time-frames can be utilized to provide the client with a frame of reference and sense of progress.

5. **Teach goal setting**. The skill of setting goals can be incorporated into therapy as a structured, formal activity similar to that used for problem solving. A simple procedure involves having the client define the *initial state* ("This is my situation now"), *goal state* ("This is what I want to be doing") and deciding on a series of steps that which lead from one to the other.

Cognitive deficits can also affect the client's access to internal verbalizations, which mediate much behavior and reduce capability to perform accurate appraisals of his emotional state and source. It is frequently difficult for clients with head injuries to get over emotions once they have been aroused, resulting in prolonged discomfort. This inability to moderate levels of emotional arousal or to attribute feelings to real situational stressors may limit the client's ability to participate in treatment. Pine (1985) has described **several techniques for use with the "fragile" patient**, which can be applied to working with the client with a brain injury:

1. **Limit the client's responses to a situation or statement made by the therapist.** It may be useful to provide a label to the client's expression of affect, and to attempt to relate the feeling to a specific source or reason (e.g., "You seem to be getting angry now. I can understand if you feel angry when we talk about your old job."
2. **Postpone dealing with difficult issues until the client's emotional state has subsided, or at points of the session where he is able to better control his emotional response.** ("Earlier we were speaking about your old job. I want to understand why that makes you angry. Let's talk about that now.")
3. **Maximize the client's preparedness and the supportive aspects of the environment.** For example, the therapist might state "I want to talk about something which may make you feel angry...listen to what I say and then we can talk about it... alright?"

An apparent lack of motivation to engage in therapy can result from the client's lack of understanding about the goals of therapy or lack of understanding or acknowledgement of their own symptoms. Neuro-behavioral problems, such as reduced initiation, poor follow-through, and difficulty formulating future-oriented goals can limit a client's capacity to be an active participant in treatment. The client's participation can be enlisted initially by using the procedures discussed above to establish agreement between client and therapist expectations. Beyond that, the therapist may adapt an attitude of active questioning, encouraging and cajoling the client to contribute his own observations, and soliciting the client's suggestions as to how to proceed with treatment. The client might be encouraged to explore the validity of symptoms or deficits, and particularly to search for similarities among situations where he has or might experience difficulty, with the therapist using what Meichenbaum (1985) refers to as the "Columbo routine of befuddlement" in order to increase a client's activity and responsibility within treatment. The client can also be encouraged to disagree with the therapist, to disprove the validity of the therapist's observations and to generate his own alternative treatment goals and directions. These procedures may temporarily increase a client's feelings of discomfort with therapy, and care needs to be taken to provide appropriate support.

Active collaboration can sometimes be achieved by incorporating some or all of the above suggestions into a procedure of *prescriptive self-monitoring*, which involves clients being asked to make specific observations and records of daily functioning outside of the treatment setting, in order to develop appropriate treatment goals. The form of self-monitoring may range from open-ended notes or a diary to specific checklists, and observations may vary from external signs of other people's reactions to clients' own personal, inner thoughts and feelings. Use of prescriptive self-monitoring can follow **several basic principles to promote the client's participation:**

1. **The client should be allowed to suggest the specific behaviors that are monitored.** In fact, the client may suggest the self-monitoring procedure itself; the therapist may merely express puzzlement over how to go about understanding what the client is all about, or confusion at the lack of behaviors appropriate for therapy, and ask the client for suggestions as to how the therapist could learn more about the client.

2. **The self-monitoring procedure should be kept simple.** The client will have better success monitoring one or two simple behaviors, than keeping track of multiple symptoms or contingencies. Less frequent intervals of monitoring (e.g., morning and evening) may be easier than hourly intervals or recordings of every occurrence.

3. **Self-monitoring of difficulties can be uncomfortable, and many clients will express some discomfort over having to note their difficulties, either because of the emotional consequences or the awkwardness of self-observation and recording.** This discomfort and difficulty should be appreciated by the therapist. It is sometimes helpful to anticipate with the client the possible discomforts as well as the difficulties in keeping up the self monitoring procedure, while encouraging the client to persist with their worthwhile endeavor.

4. Reinforce the fact that it is the client's idea that prescriptive self-monitoring be conducted, or at least that he has agreed to do so. It is also good to reinforce how helpful the information will be to the therapist and therapy. (e.g., "So, what you've come up with is a way to keep track of any times when you might get in trouble by not paying attention. You think this probably happens more with your wife than your boss, but we're not sure about that. This is great, this will really help me understand what's happening with you during the week.")

5. Use the information obtained from self-monitoring, whatever the results. Even when clients have been unable or unwilling to maintain the self-monitoring outside of sessions, or when they have not observed any difficulties, this information can be incorporated into the treatment session and developed into the treatment focus. The value of prescriptive self-monitoring lies in the facilitation of the active-collaborative role on the part of the client.

For the client who remains unable to become actively engaged in treatment, this lack of collaboration needs to be confronted within the treatment session. One of the most common errors of treatment is the failure to approach the client who presents as uninvolved in treatment. Although confrontation has sometimes acquired a negative connotation in rehabilitation, it remains an effective therapist intervention which need not be hostile or threatening. Interventions – to create a situation where the client *experiences* a discrepancy between the expected and actual level of performance, or between the therapist and client's views of treatment – may be effective in enlisting the client's active participation in the treatment process. In our opinion, there is little risk in the use of confrontation in therapy if the preliminary stages of establishing a shared set of expectancies and belief in the benevolent intentions of the therapist have been achieved. The failure to establish the client as an active participant is more detrimental to therapy than the possible negative consequences of confrontation conducted within the therapeutic relationship.

Client Commitment, Denial and Resistance

The subjective lack of appreciation for the existence or severity of deficits after injury, represents a particular area of significance for clients with head injury and will often influence greatly the client's commitment to therapy. The issue of denial is therefore of central concern to the rehabilitation counseling process. Although denial of illness has been identified as a consequence of a variety of diseases (Weinstein & Kahn, 1955), the particular concerns regarding the client with a traumatic brain injury appear predicated on the assumption that the denial process interferes with the processes of rehabilitation, psychosocial adaptation, and vocational adjustment. The patient referred for counseling who promptly denies having any problems, represents a particular source of challenge, and potential frustration, for the therapist attempting to deliver treatment. Not surprisingly, these clients may have limited ability to utilize, or benefit from, treatment. Should these clients continue to deny or minimize any problems, despite the therapist's best efforts, they may be considered to be resisting treatment. Furthermore, clients who fail to acknowledge their real limitations may assume excessive vocational or social responsibilities, fail to recognize or compensate for their errors, and have difficulty accepting assistance. Rehabilitation professionals typically assume that awareness and acknowledgement of deficits is associated with more effective treatment and better outcomes. Prigatano (1986) and others indicated that patients with better rehabilitation outcomes exhibited better emotional and motivational functioning, based on relatives' report. Fordyce and Roueche (1986) identified two groups of patients based on patient, family and staff ratings of competency prior to treatment. One group rated themselves similar to the ratings of staff, whereas the other group exhibited a pronounced tendency to underestimate their level of impairment when compared with staff members' estimations. The latter group could be further subdivided on the basis of change in patients' ratings relative to staff ratings over the course of rehabilitation. In one group, patient and staff ratings became more similar, whereas for the final group, the differences in perspective and beliefs about level of impairment actually increased. Among the patients who showed increased awareness of deficits, 78% were engaged in productive activity following their rehabilitation; but among the patients with persistent lack of awareness of deficits, only 25% were engaged in productive activity.

Clinically, these findings suggest that for clients unable to make a commitment to treatment, due to their unawareness of deficits, priority needs to be given to addressing the client's awareness deficits and resistance to therapy. A goal of counseling can be to increase the client's capacity for self-observation, which might be accomplished by providing them with specific, objective feedback and emphasizing the educative and informative aspects of therapy. The use of videotape can be effective in providing clients with feedback about their interpersonal and communication skills (Helffenstein & Wechsler, 1982). Such feedback can be repeated as required by the client to compensate for attention, memory, or comprehension deficits. In addition, repeated observations of their videotaped performance may allow the client to more objectively evaluate their own behavior. Videotapes of the clients' performance can be used to actually teach them and have them practice the skills of self-monitoring and self-assessment. For example, we have frequently used a relatively simple sensorimotor task and had clients evaluate themselves as "correct" or "incorrect" after each trial. Despite the relative simplicity of this procedure , many clients have difficulty evaluating their performance accurately. Clients are then shown a tape of another person imitating the movements, and asked to judge whether they were imitated "correctly" (i.e., the same) or "incorrectly" (i.e., differently). Next, the clients are shown the tape of themselves performing the task and asked to judge their own performance from the videotape. Finally, they are given practice in evaluating their own performance in "real time."

This same *objective self-awareness training* procedure can be utilized with tasks and work behaviors of increasing complexity. Formal checklists and behavioral self-monitoring inventories can also be incorporated into a variety of settings and adapted to review the occurrence of any number of functional or interpersonal behaviors. Given the opportunity for structured self-observation, clients' behavior will often show a reactive change in the desired direction, and this therapeutic change can be further enhanced by providing the client with feedback about the accuracy of his self-observation (Kazdin, 1974). These findings suggest that overt self-observation may compensate for the loss of internalized self-monitoring.

Another intervention for decreased awareness is the use of community based activities (e.g., work trials and situational assessments) that place the client in real-life activities, and avoid the artificiality and arbitrariness of the treatment environment. Clients can have an active role in selecting the setting and activity for such interventions, based on their previous activities or future plans. This approach typically has increased face validity and meaningfulness for many clients and may also provide salient feedback about their "real-life" performance. Additionally, this treatment approach appears to transfer some of the control of treatment from therapist to client, which can increase compliance and reduce one potential source of emotional distress. Cues from the work environment and from co-workers assist in increasing clients' self-awareness and their social awareness, and the therapist can become an ally in the absorption and adaptation processes. The use of community-based and real-life treatment environments appears to be particularly appropriate to vocational issues and can be readily incorporated into place-and-train and job coaching models of vocational rehabilitation.

Individual therapy can also be utilized with the client who exhibits denial or unawareness of deficits. Particular attention can be paid to exploring and defining the client's efficacy expectations (i.e., the client's belief that they will be able to execute specific behaviors leading to desired outcomes) (Bandura, 1977). Rather than relying on normative or dichotomous neuropsychological statements about deficits, or the therapist's performance expectancies, the client can be asked to predict his own performance capabilities. This allows the therapist to address the discrepancies between the client's perceived and actual competences.

Therapeutic interventions can be either:

(a) Verbal and evocative, emphasizing the process of accurate self-appraisal (e.g., "How sure are you that you can do that?", "Are you sure you have done that right? How sure?", "What would it mean if you're unable to do that, but you think you can?");

(b) More directive and behaviorally oriented (e.g., "You're still making more mistakes than you said were acceptable. You either have to slow down and correct your own errors...or you could change your goal. Which do you want to do?"); or

(c) A combination of both.

The possible relations and implications of the client's deficits to his everyday functioning, including any difficulty in accurately assessing their own performance, can be interpreted with them regularly. In offering such interpretations, it is preferable to challenge the *evidence* for the clients' beliefs about their functioning, rather than the beliefs themselves. In general, we agree with Deaton's (1986) suggestion that "all treatments should involve a balance between positive (supportive) and negative (confrontative) elements" (p. 235).

Within the context of a therapeutic alliance, another strategy can be to predict the client's denial. For example, a 24-year-old severely head-injured man with marked impairments in memory and executive function entered post-acute rehabilitation with pronounced denial of any disability and insistence that he could return to work. This denial appeared to represent both an inability to integrate the changes in his abilities with his self-concept due to his severe memory deficits, inability to appreciate his limitations in any abstract sense, and the need to avoid becoming emotionally overwhelmed when the deficits were made apparent to him. He rejected any affiliation with other clients, all of whom had "something wrong with their brains" and were therefore nothing like him. Instead, he fostered a strong association with the various rehabilitation therapists, whom he referred to as "teachers" who were giving him classes so that he could open his own business. He exhibited a strong identification and personalized relationship with the psychotherapist, whom he regarded as a mentor and potential business partner.

Over the course of treatment, the psychotherapist anticipated for this patient his inevitable frustration with treatment, followed by progressive mistrust and devaluation of his therapists, and his eventual disillusionment with his psychotherapist, as well. A condition of unconditional acceptance and support was maintained in psychotherapy despite other difficulties, including his expanding anger and hostility toward the treatment. At the same time, he was encouraged to participate in a process of proximal goal setting, and to identify a concrete and specific progression of steps and mediating goals which would be necessary to enable him to return to his own business. Although not all of the difficulties associated with this client's treatment were avoided, the anticipation of this client's expanding denial and emotional distress increased the therapist's credibility, allowed the client to gradually acknowledge his feelings of dependency and low self-esteem, accept some responsibility for his feelings of anger and his interpersonal problems, and revise his treatment goals without a loss of self-respect. Although, several years later, he continues to exhibit marked reductions in his social and vocational functioning, he has made continued progress in terms of his psychological adjustment and sense of self-worth.

In practice, it is often difficult to differentiate an organic lack of awareness from psychologically and emotionally based denial, or to determine the degree to which they may coexist. In addition, it is likely that the degree of premorbid characterological rigidity and defensiveness is likely to contribute to the person's ability to acknowledge deficits after a head injury. It is therefore important to obtain a thorough history and to inquire about the client's response to stressful situations, and his willingness to acknowledge problems or attribute them to psychological or personal causes. (It is worth keeping in mind that most of us will tend to attribute difficulties to an external cause; persons who don't are probably being treated for depression.)

Clinical experience suggests that clients who exhibit more extensive and severe neuropsychological deficits often show the least awareness of their disability. This would suggest an organic basis for the decreased awareness. In these cases, it is common for the client to exhibit a reduced awareness of the physical and social environment and diminished interpersonal sensitivity, along with reduced self-monitoring and self-awareness. On the other hand, complaints of disability appear to be related to increased emotional distress and psychopathology, independent of neuropsychological status. This suggests that psychological denial in some cases does represent an emotional reaction and protective response in the face of increasing recognition of disability and distress. Clients may show a normal awareness of the environment and psychological vigilance in their interpersonal functioning, while offering apparently specific and selective disclaimers regarding their objective deficits. We would propose a simple strategy, which may assist in differentiating between organic and psychological forms of unawareness: If the client is provided with increased information and objective feedback about his deficits, and his ability to acknowledge his deficits increases, then his lack of appreciation for their deficits is probably neurologically mediated. If the client is provided with specific information and evidence regarding his deficit, and there appears to be an increased resistance to acknowledging his limitations and evidence of emotional distress, he is probably exhibiting a protective emotional response.

In some cases, of course, clients should be allowed to maintain their denial, especially when it does not interfere with therapy or daily functioning. Awareness itself may not be a valuable commodity, and the need for clients to "mourn their deficits" may have more to do with therapists' values and needs than with clients' treatment. (Alexy, 1983). Therapists need to consider the client's perspective and respect his experience. In cases where the client continues to be resistant or unable to commit to therapy, he may be resisting an interpretation or treatment plan that is simply untenable or irrelevant to him.

Specific Interventions for Cognitive and Behavioral Problems Related to Vocational Rehabilitation Procedures and Outcomes

It is commonly believed that the cognitive and behavioral problems exhibited by clients with traumatic brain injury are the major obstacles to return to work. Price and Baumann (1990), for example, identified various critical work behaviors considered necessary to succeed in competitive employment. They found that vocationally related difficulties for persons with traumatic brain injury were related to these critical work behaviors rather than to specific job skills and aptitudes. Over 50% of head-injured workers had problems with work performance, which included behaviors such as exercising good social judgement and presentation. The primary reasons for poor performance in this area were:

Acceptance of Worker Role: carrying out work assignments independently, poor judgement in the use of obscenities or playing practical jokes, temperamental behavior.

Degree of Comfort with Supervisor: becoming upset when corrected.

Appropriateness of Personal Relations with Supervisor: discussing personal problems not related to work.

Social Communication Skills: expressing likes and dislikes inappropriately, expressing negative feelings inappropriately, interrupting others while speaking.

The second general dimension related to poor work performance seemed related to cognitive abilities such as learning ability and capacity for self-direction on the job. Over 40% of clients were found to have difficulty in this area of task orientation, which included the following behaviors:

Work Persistence: maintaining work pace when distractions occurred.

Amount of Supervision Required: inability to recognize their own mistakes, needing more than the average amount of supervision, requiring frequent help with problems.

Work Tolerance: inability to perform tasks that required variety, inability to accept changes in work assignments.

In general, problems with work conformance seemed to be related to social judgement and emotional control, while problems in task orientation were related to cognitive abilities such as sustaining attention, problem solving, mental flexibility, and new learning.

Stapleton, Bennett, and Parenté (1989) obtained reports and behavioral ratings from job coaches who had experience working with clients with traumatic brain injury in order to determine which behaviors were most problematic on the work site. Major problems were evident in the slow acquisition of job skills, verbal and visual memory, judgment, inflexibility of thinking, and anxiety. Moderate problems on the work site were evident in completion of work in a timely fashion, obsessive/compulsive behavior, inability to detect/correct errors, inability to work independently attention and concentration deficits, poor social interaction skills, intellectual limitations, inability to organize/prioritize tasks, difficulty staying on task in the face of distractions, inability to work without structure or make plans independently, and physical limitations.

Once again, most of these problems could be related to two areas. The first included social judgment, planning, insight and social skills, while the second area included problems in attention and concentration, memory, and new learning. Thus, there appears to be reasonable consistency between these two studies in the identification of the kinds of deficits that are most likely to impact on clients vocationally. These behaviors can serve as a basis for the rehabilitation counselor's interventions. It should be recognized that clients' deficits in these areas, especially at the stage of recovery where the client is attempting vocational re-entry, are likely to be permanent limitations. These interventions are not *remedial*, but are intended to facilitate the counseling process and perhaps assist the client to compensate for residual difficulties.

Interventions and Compensations

Learning and acquisition of new job skills. There is probably a trade-off between speed and accuracy, so that reducing the time spent on new learning may simply increase mistakes. Learning can, however, be facilitated by providing the client with specific instructions and opportunity to practice new skills. Clients may need to practice new work skills outside of the work environment, which obviously requires more time and effort. The greater the similarity between the training tasks and environment and the actual skills required on the work site, the greater the likelihood that the client will acquire and maintain skills. Overlearning through repetition will typically make the activity more routine and efficient, although such extended training may actually be detrimental if the client is going to be required to perform a variety of different activities.

It is not unusual for clients to require greater amounts of time preparing for their work, in order to compensate for the greater amount of time required to perform activities while actually on the job. When giving instructions, it is of benefit to obtain a comprehension check from the client by having them repeat or paraphrase the instructions before carrying out the activity. Delays and distractions between the client receiving the instructions and carrying out the activity should be avoided or minimized. (See Monograph #4 by Wehman, McMahon, and Fraser, 1991 for additional discussion of worker training procedures.)

Error recognition and correction. Clients might be taught to use a formal "self-checking routine" in order to detect errors. This will frequently require a step-by-step comparison between the client's actual performance and the job requirements. When an error is detected, it may be necessary for the client to perform the entire activity once again. Thus it is preferable to check progress as frequently as is feasible, throughout the activity, rather than waiting until the task is completed. Once again, the trade-off between speed and accuracy applies.

Sustained attention and resistance to distraction. It is probably most efficient to manipulate the environment to reduce distractors , whenever possible. Clients may be able to remove work from a large office or common work area in order to work on material in a relatively quiet or isolated environment. During counseling sessions, clients' ability to attend to a task can be addressed by providing them with periodic cues from the counselor. These cues can be as simple as giving them a token after a defined time period of sustained attention, or giving them a written prompt to monitor whether they have been maintaining attention. The interval of time between the counselor's providing cues can then be increased, or the client can be given more responsibility for self-monitoring of attention lapses and self-reinforcement for paying attention. These procedures of using a reinforcer or written cue to maintain attention to a task can be readily incorporated into the work setting, with the supervisor or job coach providing cues as necessary.

Attention to task can also be increased by providing benefits to staying on task. For example, the tokens used as cues can be given either symbolic or tangible value. On the work site, the client can also be reinforced for maintaining on-task behavior by being provided periodic benefits to being on-task. For example, work breaks can be made contingent on task-performance rather than time contingencies.

Problem solving and organization. Clients can utilize some form of formal problem solving framework (e.g., D'Zurilla & Goldfried, 1971) which systematically directs the client through a series of cognitive stages. These stages typically include the identification of the problem, review of alternative solutions, selection of a response, and verification of a solution. This procedure is well suited to training interpersonal problem solving within the context of therapy using a variety of social, functional and vocational examples (Foxx, Martella, & Marchand-Martella, 1989). It also appears effective to have clients identify potential or actual problems from their daily experience, and to address these within the problem solving session.

This procedure may have particular utility in the context of counseling the client about job options, or it may be expanded to involve the client in the discussion and evaluation of specific work behaviors and interpersonal behaviors on the work site. Particular attention can be given to having the client identify both the short term and long term *costs* and *benefits* to a particular "solution", as well as considering both the personal and social costs and benefits.

Completion of work in a timely fashion and ability to carry out work without prompts or excess supervision. Self-management techniques and checklists may be taught to increase a client's independence and ability to perform on a regular schedule. For example, Shafer (1987) used a self-instructional procedure with a client who had difficulty completing a series of janitorial tasks independently. This procedure involved four steps: asking questions of himself about what tasks need to be completed; answering the questions in the form of a rehearsed series of statements; guiding the performance with follow-up statements related to individual task analyses and requirements; and self-reinforcement with praising statements. The same procedure can be supported with written prompts, checklists, visual graphs, portable tape recordings of the self-statements, or other cues to support clients cognitive functioning.

Social judgement and communication. Inappropriate social behaviors and poor social judgement may be related to lack of knowledge of or ability to perform necessary social skills; lack of awareness about ones' own behavior; difficulty recognizing social cues and feedback; or reduced behavioral self-control. Clients should be given immediate, direct feedback regarding their social interactions within the counseling session, and therapists are obviously a powerful model for appropriate social behavior. It is important to assess the client's available social skills as a possible source of poor work behavior. For example, one woman was frequently late or absent from her job without notifying her supervisor, who became increasingly irritated by her lack of respect and "not caring" about her job. In counseling, she appeared motivated and cooperative, valued her work experience, and recognized the difficulties that her poor attendance was causing. She revealed that her transportation was often delayed in picking her up, but did not know what to do when that happened. As an interim intervention, at least, the client was taught to notify her supervisor by phone whenever her ride was more than 15 minutes late.

Role playing can be used to develop a repertoire of appropriate social responses. It is often helpful for the patient to have a sample of well-practiced and routine responses for different social situations, e.g., greeting and responding to supervisors and co-worker; waiting for appropriate moments to speak or making nondisruptive interruptions; responding to suggestions or criticisms; and so on. Having a rehearsed selection of responses will often reduce social anxiety and help to avoid the emotional consequences of difficult social interactions, as well. Inappropriate social behaviors may be related to difficulty in understanding the intentions or meanings of others' actions. Clients can practice forming "interpersonal hypotheses" to explain the behavior of others, and validate these with the therapist (Leftoff, 1983). Self-monitoring of inappropriate verbalizations or social behaviors can be conducted through diaries, notebooks or checklist and can be an effective means of providing the client with feedback about his or her behavior and training social skills. The majority of problems with social and work behaviors exhibited by clients with traumatic brain injury are probably related to their cognitive and behavioral deficits resulting from the injury, rather than being intrapsychic or conflict-based. Treatment, therefore, needs to assist clients to recognize and compensate for their deficits in order to reduce these symptoms.

Group Work and Group Therapy

Group psychotherapy can be a valuable component of counseling for clients with traumatic brain injury, and may be especially valuable in facilitating the process of socialization by which the client learns to relate with others and assume roles within the family, community and society (Diehl, 1984). Group therapy provides a means to place the client in a social situation, and therefore more closely approximate the demands of real life. This can serve to reduce clients' social isolation, and at the same time demands a broader repertoire of social and inter-personal behaviors. The group situation can be an effective means of having clients experience the effects of their injury on their social behavior, and the effects of their social behavior on others. Within the group, socially appropriate behavior needs to be maintained while inappropriate behaviors are diminished. Experience with group pro-cesses of turn-taking, compromise, personal risk-taking, self-disclosure and other social skills are readily transferred to work and daily living situations. The use of structured exercises, homework assignments, and videotaped feedback are applicable in the group setting, and can be of assistance in helping clients to develop awareness and ensuring that generalization of skills or behaviors is actually occurring.

For some clients, sharing experiences with other persons who have traumatic brain injury is a powerful form of alleviating the sense of alienation and demoralization. Clients may particularly benefit from feedback from other clients regarding their cognitive limitations, emo-tional reactions, and social behaviors. In many instances, clients are able to accept this peer feedback when they are unable or unwilling to accept feedback from a professional or others. Support groups may be structured around specific vocational issues, e.g., job seeking or job placement. For clients who seem unable to appreciate or tolerate group process, it is possible to have more structured, psychoeducational or "discussion groups" in which clients can ask questions about specific medical, neuropsychological, vocational, or other factual topics. This can be effective in promoting a gradual expression and sharing of clients' experiences and feelings.

Clemmons and Fraser (1991) have identified a format for group work with clients with traumatic brain injury, that contains four aspects. These are: a climate of acceptance, a bridge to reality, a sharing of the patients world, and a climate of appreciation. This basic model of group interaction is important in the development of a positive attitude toward group interaction by both clients and counselors, and may be seen as a precursor to developing the therapeutic conditions discussed by Yalom (1975). In using group interactions to foster vocational activities, there may be a combination of psychoeducational, behavior change, and support group emphases. According to Fraser, the utility of group interaction to the vocational re-entry process includes the following:

1. Reinforcement of program goals
2. Evaluation of social functioning
3. Opportunity to evaluate a spouse, parent or friend as a resource
4. Presentation of didactic information regarding head injury and related issues
5. Building an "*esprit de corps*," reviewing the progress of different group members within the vocational program
6. Specific problem-solving within a job-related context

The format and content of these groups appear to work well with clients, spouses, parents and friends included in the group. This type of group requires an active and well-organized therapist. In some instances, separate groups for clients and significant others may allow difficult emotional issues to be more readily addressed.

Prigatano (1986) and others have utilized cognitive group therapy and group psychotherapy, as well as an ancillary educational group for relatives of clients. Cognitive group therapy is a form of group therapy that focuses on improving social perception and facilitating effective communication. Initially, the purpose of the group is to increase the level of self-awareness of cognitive strengths and weaknesses. It is the responsibility of group members to provide appropriate feedback to one another. This process frequently generates strong emotional reactions, but is necessary to help individuals form realistic perceptions and expectations.

Group psychotherapy, as utilized by Prigatano's group, is a more traditional therapy directed at the emotional and motivational disturbances associated with brain injury. The focus is on helping clients to recognize and modify the various types of personality and affective disturbances which are associated with traumatic brain injury. The initial aim of group psychotherapy is to help clients break down their sense of social isolation, and to help them identify their emotional difficulties. A long-term aim is to have clients be able to identify their own emotional reactions in a group setting and to deal with these collectively in a productive way. It may be helpful to have a prepared list of topics for discussion at different sessions. These might include what group psychotherapy is all about, common emotional reactions and personality changes after brain injury, the catastrophic reaction, body image, self confidence, and feelings concerning work and going back to work at a lower level (Prigatano, 1986). Mangel (1990) has developed a structured format for group psychotherapy based on the various topics suggested by Prigatano (1986) and others, which includes a framework for facilitating client discussion and feedback.

Conclusions

In general, it is wise to consider the counseling relationship as a model of clients' interactions with the rest of their social and vocational environment. The therapist needs to be sensitive to a client's cognitive, behavioral and emotional limitations and adjust the counseling interactions accordingly, while maintaining an attitude of caring and empathic understanding. The therapist also needs to be able to confront the client, to challenge the client, and to foster the prospect for change; acceptance of the client does not mean acceptance of all of the client's behaviors.

The therapist also needs to be able to promote the application of skills and behaviors outside of the treatment session. The functional application of therapy appears to be enhanced when training is prolonged, the client is given increasing responsibility for his behavior, and feedback about the utility and appropriate application of his behavior is provided. The failure to maintain an appropriate "therapeutic distance" constitutes a common therapeutic error. When addressing the clients cognitive deficits we have relied on a simple rule: when the client succeeds, provide less assistance; when the client fails, provide more assistance. In similar fashion, when the client appears to have difficulty engaging or participating in therapy, the therapist needs to approach the client and increase the client's involvement within therapy; when the client appears to be over-reliant on the therapist and has difficulty in applying the lessons of therapy outside of the treatment environment, the therapist needs to increase the client's autonomy and involvement outside of treatment.

If the return to work does represent a "return to normality" for clients who have sustained traumatic brain injury, then the therapeutic relationship and interactions represent a powerful vehicle for that return. Together they provide clients with opportunities for new learning and experiencing, for developing awareness about their presumed and actual abilities, for confronting – and hopefully reducing – the discrepancies between their assumptive world and their daily reality.

References

Alexy, W. D. (1983). Perceptions of deficits following brain injury: A reply to Roueche and Fordyce. *Cognitive Rehabilitation, 1:4,* 23.

Bandura, L. (1977). Self-efficacy: Toward a unifying theory of behavior. *Psychology Review, 84,* 191-215.

Beutler, L. E., & Clarkin J. F. (1990). *Systematic treatment selection.* New York: Bruner/Mazel.

Chelune, G. J., Heaton, R. K., & Lehman, R. A. (1986). Relation of neuropsychological and personality test results to patients' complaints of disability. In G. Goldstein, & R. Tarter (Eds.), *Advances in Clinical Neuropsychology (Vol. 3).* New York: Plenum Press.

Cicerone, K. D. (1989). Psychotherapeutic interventions with traumatically brain-injured patients. *Rehabilitation Psychology, 34,* 105-114.

Cicerone, K. D. (1987). *Overcoming obstacles to change.* Presented at National Head Injury Foundation Sixth Annual Symposium, San Diego, CA.

Clemmons, D. C., & Fraser, R. T. (1991). *Vocational re-entry of the traumatic brain injured: A demonstration.* Unpublished manuscript, University of Washington, Department of Neurological Surgery, Seattle.

Crosson, B., Barco, P. P., Velozo, C. A., Bolesta, M. M., Cooper, P. V., Werts, D., & Brobeck, T. C. (1989). Awareness and compensation in post-acute head injury rehabilitation. *Journal of Head Trauma Rehabilitation, 4,* 46-54.

Deaton, A. V. (1986). Denial in the aftermath of traumatic head injury: Its manifestations, measurement, and treatment. *Rehabilitation Psychology, 31,* 231-240.

Diehl, L. (1984). Patient-family education. In M. Rosenthal, E. R. Griffith, M. Bond, & J. R. Miller (Eds.), *Rehabilitation of the Head Injured Adult.* Philadelphia: F.A. Davis.

Dunbar, J. (1980). Adhering to medical advice: A review. *International Journal of Mental Health, 9,* 70-87.

D'Zurilla, T. J., & Goldfried, M. R. (1971). Problem solving and behavior modification. *Journal of Abnormal Psychology, 78*, 107-126.

Faust, P., Guilmette, T. J., Hart, K., Arkes, H. R., Fishburne, F. J., & Davey, L. (1988). Neuropsychologist's training, experience, and judgement accuracy. *Archives of Clinical Neuropsychology, 3*, 145-163.

Fordyce, D. J., & Roueche, J. R. (1986). Changes in perspectives of disability among patients, staff, and relatives during rehabilitation of brain injury. *Rehabilitation Psychology, 31*, 217-229.

Foxx, R. M., Martella, R. C., & Marchand-Martella, N. E. (1989). The acquisition, maintenance, and generalization of problem-solving skills by closed head injured adults. *Behavior Therapy, 20*, 61-76.

Galano, J. (1977). Treatment effectiveness as a function of client involvement in goal-setting and goal-planning. *Goal Attainment Review, 3*, 1-8.

Helffenstein, D. A., & Wechsler, F. (1982). The use of Interpersonal Process Recall (IPR) in the remediation of interpersonal and communication skill deficits in the newly brain injured. *Clinical Neuropsychology, 4*, 139-143.

Kazdin, N. (1974). Reactive self-monitoring: The effects of response desirability, goal setting, and feedback. *Journal of Consulting and Clinical Psychology, 42*, 704-716.

Leftoff, S. (1983). Psychopathology in the light of brain injury: A case study. *Journal of Clinical Neuropsychology, 5*, 51-63.

Lobitz, C., & Shephard, K. (1983). Effect of compatibility on goal-achievement in patient physical therapist dyads. *Physical Therapy, 63*, 319-324.

Mangel, H. (1990). *Structured group psychotherapy with patients with traumatic brain injury.* Presented at Rebuilding Shattered Lives: Third Annual Conference on Traumatic Brain Injury, Woodbridge, New Jersey.

Meichenbaum, D. (1985). *Stress Inoculation Training.* New York: Pergamon.

Pepping, M., & Roueche, J.R. (1990). Psychosocial consequences of significant brain injury. In D. E. Tupper, & K. D. Cicerone (Eds.), *The neuropsychology of everyday life: Issues in development and rehabilitation.* Boston:Kluwer Academic.

Pine, F. (1985). *Developmental theory and clinical process.* New Haven: Yale University Press.

Price, P., & Baumann, W. L. (1990). Working: The key to normalization after brain injury. In D. E. Tupper & K. D.Cicerone (Eds.), *The neuropsychology of everyday life: Issues in development and rehabilitation.* Boston: Kluwer Academic.

Prigatano, G. (1986). *Neuropsychological rehabilitation after brain injury.* Baltimore: The Johns Hopkins University Press.

Shafer, M. S. (1987). Supported competitive employment: The use of self-management programming in the follow-along process. *Journal of Rehabilitation,* July/August/September, 331-36.

Stapleton, M., Bennet, P., & Parenté, R. (1989). Job coaching traumatically brain injured individuals: Lessons learned. *Cognitive Rehabilitation, 7,* 18-21.

Weinstein, E. A., & Kahn, R. L. (1955). *Denial of illness.* Springfield, IL: Charles C. Thomas.

Yalom, I. (1975). *Theory and practice of group psychotherapy.* New York: Basic Books.